Table of Contents

Introduction

FLOUR, WATER, SALT, AND YEAST—these four simple ingredients when combined create the magic that is bread. Baking bread is a time-honored tradition honed over more than six thousand years. The craft is a truly sensory experience: the warmth of the dough in your hands, the aromas lingering in the air during baking, the crackling of the crust as it cools, the complex and seductive flavors on your tongue. Yet for some, the process of making bread strikes fear in their hearts. I hope to change that.

In the world of bread bakers and grammarians alike, there has been much debate about the usage of the word artisan. Artisan is actually a noun that refers to a skilled worker or craftsman, but due to the ebbs and flows of popular usage, it is applied as an adjective for carefully handcrafted food and beverages, such as cheese, wine, chocolate, and, of course, bread. The romance associated with something handmade, especially in our hustle-bustle world, entices people to seek out artisan products. Unfortunately, the word artisan is sometimes liberally used and abused in the marketing campaigns of larger bakeries and corporations, diluting its meaning.

As for defining artisan, if you asked fifty artisan bakers to describe exactly what being an artisan baker means, fifty different styles would be conjured. My personal definition of artisan bread is handmade bread that is crafted using quality, natural ingredients and does not include any added chemicals or artificial ingredients. Anyone who considers himself an artisan baker has the responsibility of aiming to reclaim the true origins of the word through experience and education.

This book contains information on Artisan sourdough cookbooks.

Artisan in food

Artisan made food is made using quality ingredients and methods that are best for the quality of the product. Classing a food as “artisan-made” declares a stamp of quality that the product is of the uppermost standards. The use of additives or improvers is usually replaced with natural ingredients and highly skilled methods of production.

Due to a large amount of manual effort and skill required to make artisan food, there are few mass-market producers. Artisan foods are expensive to produce in mass and due to being additive-free will have a shorter shelf life. As artisanal foods cost a high price to produce most are sold locally in farmers markets or delis.

Artisan bread

The word “artisan” gets thrown around a lot these days. There’s everything from artisan pasta to artisan umbrellas. A lot of the time, the term doesn’t add much to the product.

However, this type of bread is substantially different from the industrially-processed loaves you might be familiar with. And there are good reasons to know the difference between them.

In this post, you'll find a comprehensive primer on artisan bread baking and the types of it.

While there's no strict definition for what makes a bread "artisan," there are some standards that artisan bread bakers typically adhere to. For the most part, they're far better-tasting and have a much more pleasing texture and aroma than industrially produced ones.

Mass-produced bread has to meet flavor standards that appeal to the largest number of people. It also needs to be reproducible and use resources as efficiently as possible. On the other hand, artisan bread is handmade with a more traditional process. The gasses, dough pressure, timing, and ingredients aren't as minutely controlled.

While making it, you don't need to use dough conditioners and low protein-count flours. Its worth noting that there are no strict standards so different bakers might use different ingredients.

Country loaves, sourdough, ciabatta, brioche, and some seeded bread are often made using artisan techniques.

Artisan Bread vs. Regular Bread

That takes care of the definition, but it doesn't explain how it's different from ordinary bread.

The main distinguishing feature between the two is consistency. Every loaf of Wonder Bread you buy will have the same flavor and texture. Since artisan bread bakers use a less controlled process, every bread will have its character and mouthfeel.

Artisan bread also typically uses traditional yeast fermenting techniques. The benefit of using traditional techniques is more flavorful bread and it often has a more nuanced flavor profile than their mass-produced counterparts. However, if you're used to the blander and more predictable taste of bread, you might go through a transitional period before you get used to the artisan one.

In mass-produced bread, there is very little fermentation built into the process which results in a more closed-cell structure. Artisan bread, on the other hand, often has a much more open and airy look to it since the bread rises from fermentation rather than the kneading process.

Note that this doesn't make artisan bread necessarily healthier. Research into the health effects of both hasn't provided any clinically significant benefits from eating artisan bread over other types of commercial ones.

Lastly, all that fermentation, careful attention, and work by hand take a lot of time. This type of bread takes far longer to make than industrialized one and consequently tends to be more expensive.

What is different in artisan bread production?

The biggest difference in artisan bread production is the amount of time used to develop the dough. To allow for extended natural fermentation the dough must be kept at a lower temperature than non-artisan made bread. Other differences include;

- Higher water content
- The use of preferment dough
- Less reliance on machinery in production

How to create different types of artisan bread

Changing the dough's ingredients or the techniques used to produce it such as the mixing time, shaping, water hydration, fermentation time or the temperature change the behavior of the dough. Different behaviors form personalized textures and flavor in the dough to create multiple bread types. A skilled baker is able to adapt dough to make several variations of bread from the same mix.

Types of Artisan Bread

Just about every recipe will have an artisan variation. Bread made with or without a pan or proofing basket can be considered artisan. The type of bread is not important in artisan classification, the ingredients selected and the methods used are what is evaluated for the term to be applied. Popular artisan bread types include:

Baguette

Best consumed within a few hours of baking this iconic french bread is one of the most popular breads found worldwide. French bread law protects the integrity of the ingredients used to make baguettes. The invention of the steam oven and the post-war working restrictions imposed after the Second World War by the French government were perfectly timed for the baguette. A quick to make bread that can be enjoyed at any occasion led the baguette to popularity in Paris and quickly adopted across the world. Be careful of bread that is described as "French Stick" or "French Bread" as these are not real baguettes!

Sourdough

Allowing time and temperature to develop the natural yeasts in the environment and raise the bread is not a new idea. The widespread use of commercial yeast nearly lost this artisan bread. The lactobacillus starter not only raises the bread, but it also matures the flour to create a dough which is easy to handle and packed full of flavour. Sourdough bread can have a very distinctive, sour and tangy taste due to the lactic acid that is produced by the starter. Here's my sourdough bread recipe for beginners to help you get started.

Focaccia

Fantastically unique bread that contains an open yet irregular crumb topped with a selection of Italian inspired toppings. The focaccia can be thin, or thick and can be sliced to make a sandwich or eaten on its own.

Rye Bread

Rye bread is high in fiber and has an extremely strong flavor when compared to other flours. A lack of gluten in rye flour can often lead to a dense, heavy bread. Combining rye and white flour is a common method that is used to make great tasting bread. The color of the rye decides how dense or dark the bread will be.

Brioche

Brioche has a rich texture due to containing copious amounts of butter and eggs. It is usually sweetened with sugar too. Brioche is eaten in France for breakfast or during the day with coffee. The most popular form is Brioche à Tête, yet brioche can be found in a loaf form too.

Ciabatta

The literal meaning of the word Ciabatta is slipper which it derives its name from. An Italian white bread used to make sandwiches usually but can be served with dinner. A properly made

Sourdough

Sourdough has always seemed like specialty bread to me. Little did I know it would almost beat out no-knead artisan bread in its easiness. And that it's amazingly delicious. And that there were health benefits of sourdough.

The idea of bread being sour totally grossed me out and I purposely stayed away from it for nearly all my life. It wasn't until I ordered a sandwich on sourdough a few years ago that I experienced the amazingly light and delicious tang of sourdough. Grilled with butter, topped with ham and melted swiss.

Sourdough is a bread made from the natural occurring yeast and bacteria in flour. In traditional sourdough recipes, you'll find three ingredients: sourdough starter (which consists of flour and water), salt and flour. There is no yeast, no milk, no oils and no sweeteners. It's about as natural as you get when it comes to bread.

What makes Sourdough special

Ask anyone who's eaten sourdough and they'll tell you that the tang is what makes it special. I agree, and in fact the signature tartness of sourdough bread comes from the same bacteria that gives yogurt and sour cream their pucker too. It's found naturally in wheat flour, along with yeast, and comes to life when the flour is mixed with water. Here's a very simple explanation of the process:

• wheat flour + water –> natural enzymes break down starches into glucose (sugar)

• natural bacteria (tang) + glucose –> food for natural yeast

• natural yeast + food –> natural leaven (carbon dioxide

• natural leaven + more flour + more water –> more natural leaven

So basically you start with flour and water. Nature takes its course and over time, you have a mixture that contains enough leaven (yeast) to make bread rise. Who knew doing so little could yield such an amazing result

Benefits of Sourdough

You guys know the health benefits of yogurt and kefir, right? Imagine those benefits, fresh and warm from the oven and smeared with butter.

Lactobacillus

Lactobacillus is the good bacteria in yogurt, kefir, sour cream, buttermilk, etc. It ferments the flour/water mixture and creates lactic acid, a catalyst that greatly increases the micronutrient profile. In simple terms, all those nutrients found in whole wheat flour are bigger and badder, and now your body is better able to use them too.

The fermentation process alone is great for your digestive system. The Lactobacillus helps feed the good bacteria found in your digestive system so they can continue to fight off the bad guys. And remember that a healthy gut means healthy body. Most of your immune system is found in your digestive system.

Phytates

One neat thing to the long soaking required of sourdough is that it breaks down much of the phytates that bind the awesome minerals in grains. With the phytates gone, our bodies can grab those nutrients and actually use them!

With those nutrients readily available, digestion of the starch is much easier on your body. In fact, the natural bacteria working with the natural yeast predigests the starch a little bit for you. The benefits of sourdough will make your tummy happy.

Remember how the natural yeast feeds on the glucose? With a large portion of the glucose devoured in the fermentation process, sourdough doesn't cause a spike in your blood sugars like processed white breads often do. The long process also breaks down many of the gluten proteins into amino acids, possibly making sourdough bread tolerable for those who are sensitive to gluten!

One last neat tid-bit: sourdough bread is less likely to stale, retains much of its moisture as it ages, and its acidity helps prevent the growth of mold! Now this doesn't mean your sourdough won't ever go stale and will never grow mold. But it's nice to know that the artisan loaf you treated yourself to at the farmer's market won't go bad too quickly.

Making it yourself

Besides the fact that most "whole wheat" breads are just really made with plain 'ol white flour, making sourdough is probably the absolute easiest homemade bread I've ever made. In fact, it nearly ties kefir for the easiest fermentation ever.

- Mix flour and water.

- Wait.
- Repeat.

The only downside of sourdough bread is that it does take time. The work itself isn't hard, but you must plan ahead if you want to make sourdough 100% from scratch. It takes a full seven days if you're using only flour and water. However, there are kits you can buy that will produce sourdough starters in as little as three days.

Cultures for Health offers several to choose from, including rye, Italian, French, whole wheat and even brown rice for those who can't take any chances with gluten. I tested out the San Francisco variety and it was almost too easy to ferment. I've already made two batches of pancakes and biscuits with the extras!

Which leads me to the goods news – once you get in the routine of feeding your starter, you're more likely to find yourself needing to use up extra starter. And once you have a starter, you can feed it more or less depending on how soon or not soon you need a certain amount

Recipes

Authentic Sourdough Sandwich Bread

Ingredients:

- 830 g all-purpose flour or bread flour
- 90 g whole-wheat flour
- 690 g water
- 20 g salt
- 184 g leaven

Directions:

Day One: Leaven Day

Before bedtime, build your leaven. Weigh 100 grams of lukewarm water in a mason jar and add 50 grams of your healthy, active starter, which you fed this morning (8-12 hours ago). Don't use freshly fed starter, it is not mature enough.

- Swirl the jar to incorporate the starter. Add 50 grams whole wheat flour and 50 grams white flour (all-purpose or bread flour). Stir with a butter knife or spatula until mixed well. Make sure no dry flour remains.

- Place the lid lightly on the jar – don't screw it on! – leave on the counter to ferment overnight.

Day Two: Mix Day

- Place your mixing bowl on the scale and weigh 640g of the water (save 50g) and 184g of your leaven. Using your hand, incorporate the leaven a bit by squeezing it through your fingers. Use the rest of your leaven in discard recipes, or simply throw away.

• Add both flours and mix together with your hand. Mix until you don't see any more dry flour in the bowl. The dough will become sticky, so it's useful to keep one hand clean. Dunk your clean hand in water, and remove the sticky dough from your other hand. Then dip your dough spatula in water and scrape the edges of the bowl, making it as clean as possible.

• Cover the bowl with a clean kitchen towel or plastic and let the dough rest for 30 minutes. This is called the autolyse, which allows the flours to absorb the water, activating the enzymes which begins the gluten development. This step is critical and cannot be rushed.

• After the autolyse, sprinkle the salt over the dough and then add the remaining 50g of water. Poke your fingers into the dough to press some salt deep inside, then fold over itself about a dozen times or so to incorporate the salt. Cover the bowl again; the bulk fermentation has begun. Set your timer for 30 minutes.

• The bulk fermentation takes four hours. During the first two hours of the bulk fermentation, the dough must be folded four times, or every 30 minutes. This is similar to kneading but is much gentler to preserve the natural gases that become captured in the dough, and is much easier on the baker.

• To fold the dough, first imagine your bowl as a compass: the edge furthest from you is north, the right edge is east, the closest edge to you is south, and the left edge is west. Dip your hand in water and reach under the dough at the east point. Grabbing it gently but firmly, pull the dough out to the east and then fold it over itself toward the west. Rotate the bowl a quarter-turn, and repeat. Do this for each "corner" of your compass, then cover with a kitchen towel. These are called stretch-and-folds.

• Set your timer for 30 minutes, and repeat the process three more times.

• Your dough now gets to rest, covered and untouched, for 1 1/2 – 2 hours. During this time, flavor and strength is developed, so don't rush this step.

• After the bulk fermentation, pull all the dough onto a floured work surface using a dough spatula. With your bench knife, cut the dough into two even pieces.

• The pieces now need to be pre-shaped. Working with one piece at a time pull the west side of the dough out and fold it toward the east. Then pull the east side out and fold it over and toward the west. Then grab the north side and fold it up toward the south, then roll the dough loosely toward the south and let rest on its seam. Do the same for the remaining piece, then lightly dust both with flour and cover with a kitchen towel. This prevents a skin from forming on the outside of the dough. Let rest for 30 minutes. This is called the bench rest.

• For the final shaping, care must be taken not to deflate the dough. Gently rub off any excess flour – the top of the dough will become the inside of the loaf, so you don't want any extra flour inside. First, gently pull out on the corners to make a very rough rectangle of dough. Just as in the pre-shaping, pull the west side of the dough out and fold it toward the east. Then pull the east side out and fold it over and toward the west. Stretch the north side up and fold down toward the south, then roll the dough down like you're rolling a yoga mat. You will hear and feel gas bubbles popping; this is okay. Repeat for the remaining piece.

• Lightly grease each bread pan with olive oil or butter, and place each dough roll into the pans. Now begins the final rise. Cover with plastic or place in a grocery bag, and put both pans into the refrigerator overnight. This is called cold-proofing. The plastic is used to prevent fridge odors from absorbing into the dough. The dough will continue to ferment slowly. You can leave your dough in the fridge for up to 48 hours, but I recommend baking around 18 hours if possible.

Day Three: Bake Day
In the morning, create a steam tray. Place two or three old kitchen towels in a cookie sheet and soak them under the faucet, filling the pan about halfway up with water. Place your steam tray on the lowermost rack of the oven and preheat at 400*F for at least 30 minutes. Keep an eye on the level of water in your steam tray. If the water boils dry, your towels will burn. To add more water, use hot tap water and pour from a watering can or a large pitcher.

• When your oven is preheated and steamed, pull the bread from the refrigerator and remove the plastic. Brush the tops with egg white if you'd like a softer, dark brown crust. Add poppy seeds, rolled oats, or any other toppings on the egg wash if desired. Place bread pans in oven and bake uncovered with steam for 20 minutes.

• After 20 minutes, carefully remove the steam tray and vent the oven. Rotate your bread pans 180*, then bake 30-35 minutes more.

• Remove the bread from their pans by tipping upside down, then place loaf directly on oven rack and bake for 5 minutes more.

• Remove and allow to cool for at least two hours. Slice and enjoy!

High-Elevation Sourdough Bread

Ingredients:

• 200 grams Leaven

• 700 grams Warm water (80°F) reserve 50g

• 900 grams All-purpose flour or bread flour

• 100 grams Whole wheat flour

• 22 grams Salt

Directions:

Day One: Leaven Day

• Before bedtime, build your leaven. Weigh 100 grams of lukewarm water in a mason jar and add 50 grams of your healthy, active starter, which you fed this morning (8-12 hours ago). Don't use freshly fed starter, it is not mature enough.

• Screw the lid on the jar and shake to incorporate the starter. Open your jar and add 50 grams whole wheat flour and 50 grams white flour (all-purpose or bread flour). Stir with a butter knife or spatula until all flour is incorporated.

• Place the lid lightly on the jar – don't screw it on, and leave on the counter to ferment overnight.

Day Two: Mix Day

• Place your mixing bowl on the scale and weigh 650g of the water and 200g of your leaven. Using your hand, incorporate the leaven a bit by squeezing it through your fingers. Save the rest of your leaven as discard to use in discard recipes, if desired.

• Add both flours and mix dough together with your hand. Mix until you don't see any more dry flour in the bowl. The dough will become sticky, so it's useful to keep one hand clean. Dunk your clean hand in water, and remove the sticky dough from your other hand. Then dip your dough spatula in water and scrape the edges of the bowl, making it as clean as possible.

• Cover the bowl with a clean kitchen towel or plastic and let the dough rest for 30 minutes. This is called the autolyse, which allows the flours to absorb the water, activating the enzymes which begins the gluten development. This step is critical and cannot be rushed.

• After the autolyse, sprinkle the salt over the dough and then add the remaining 50g of water. Poke your fingers into the dough to press some salt deep inside, then fold over itself about a dozen times or so to incorporate the salt. Cover the bowl again; the bulk fermentation has begun. Set your timer for 20 minutes.

• The high-elevation bulk fermentation takes 2.5 – 3 hours. During the first two hours of the bulk fermentation, the dough must be folded six times, or every 20 minutes. This is similar to kneading but is much gentler to preserve the natural gases that become captured in the dough, and is much easier on the baker. It's also two extra folds than a regular sourdough recipe, but within the same time period.

• To fold the dough, first imagine your bowl as a compass: the edge furthest from you is north, the right edge is east, the closest edge to you is south, and the left edge is west. Dip your hand in water and reach under the dough at the east point. Grabbing it gently but firmly, pull the dough out to the east and then fold it over itself toward the west. Rotate the bowl a quarter-turn, and repeat. Do this for each "corner" of your compass, then cover with a kitchen towel.

• Set your timer for 20 minutes, and repeat the process five more times.

• Your dough now gets to rest, covered and untouched, for 30-60 minutes. During this time, flavor and strength is developed, so don't rush this step. However, this is where over-fermentation can occur, so the higher your elevation, the shorter this period should be. I live at 5,700 feet and I usually let my dough rest for 45 minutes.

• After the bulk fermentation, pull all the dough onto a floured work surface using a dough spatula. With your bench knife, cut the dough into three even pieces. Scrape the bench knife under one piece, and move it away from the other.

• The pieces now need to be pre-shaped. Working with one piece at a time, pull the west side of the dough out and fold it toward the east. Then pull the east side out and fold it over and toward the west. Rotate your dough 90°, and repeat. Do the same for the remaining piece(s), then lightly dust with flour and cover with a kitchen towel. This prevents a skin from forming on the outside of the dough. Let rest for 30 minutes. This is called the bench rest.

• For the final shaping, care must be taken not to deflate the dough. Gently rub off any excess flour – the top of the dough will become the inside of the loaf, so you don't want any extra flour inside. Just as in the pre-shaping, pull the west side of the dough out and fold it toward the east. Then pull the east side out and fold it over and toward the west. Rotate your dough 90°, and repeat. Flip the loaf so it is seam side down on your work surface, and using both hands, twist the dough as you tuck it under itself.

There are great YouTube videos with different techniques for this, but the goal is the same: to increase the surface tension without tearing the dough. You'll feel the dough tighten as you do this. Repeat for the remaining piece.

• Line your proofing baskets or medium-size bowls with basket liners or clean linen kitchen towels. Lightly dust them with rice flour (all-purpose flour isn't as good as rice flour for this job, but it could work if that's all you heave – use it generously!), covering the sides and bottom. This prevents the dough from sticking when you flip it out. Lift each piece of dough with the bench knife and flip it gently into the basket, so the seams are facing up.

• Now begins the final rise. You can cover the loaves and leave them on the counter for 3-4 hours if you'd like to bake today. However, what I recommend is using your refrigerator to slow the final rise so you can bake in the morning. This is called cold-proofing. To do this, slide each basket into their own plastic grocery or produce bag, and place in the fridge overnight. The plastic is used to prevent fridge odors from absorbing into the dough, and to prevent a skin from forming on the dough. The dough will continue to ferment over the next 8-12 hours.

Day Three: Bake Day

• In the morning, put your baking vessel and lid in the oven and preheat to 500°F. It's ideal to let your oven sit at 500°F for 30-40 minutes beyond the preheating phase, so your baking vessel is screaming hot. When it's ready, remove a basket from the fridge.

• Take a minute to get your things ready: Prepare a square of parchment paper on a thin cutting board, bring the flour close by, and have your bread lame (or razor blade) ready to go.

• Place the parchment square on the basket, place your hand on top, and gently flip the dough out into your hand. Place the dough on the cutting board. Dust the dough with flour and lightly rub it around the sides and top.

• Holding the lame at a 45° angle, score your loaf. This takes practice. Hold the cutting board with one hand as you slice the furthest corner of the blade into the dough. The easiest and most effective scores are a deep line about an inch or two from the bottom, running half the circumference of the dough, or a simple square. See my post on Scoring Techniques.

• Wearing heavy duty oven mitts, pull out your oven rack and remove the lid from your baking vessel. Working quickly but carefully, transfer the dough into the pan by holding the cutting board over it and pulling on the parchment. Replace the lid, reduce the oven temperature to 475°F, and set the timer for 30 minutes.

• When the time is up, carefully remove the lid from the pan and continue baking uncovered for 15 minutes.

• When the loaf is done, transfer it to a wire cooling rack. If you don't have one, tip it on its side so air can circulate around the bottom. To test doneness, knock on the bottom of the loaf: it should sound hollow. Allow it to cool for at least an hour or two before slicing so it can cool completely. Hot bread does not slice well.

• Set the oven temperature back to 500°F, and put both pieces of your baking vessel back in the oven. Let these heat for 10 minutes, then repeat above steps for your other basket of dough. Congratulations, you just made sourdough at elevation!

Sourdough Cinnamon Crumb Cake

Ingredients:

Topping

• 2 cups (241g) King Arthur Unbleached All-Purpose Flour

• 1 cup (198g) granulated sugar

• 1 1/2 teaspoons cinnamon

• 1/2 teaspoon salt

• 1 teaspoon vanilla extract

• 1/2 teaspoon almond extract

• 12 tablespoons (170g) unsalted butter, melted

Batter

• 8 tablespoons (113g) unsalted butter, at room temperature, at least 65°F

• 1 cup (198g) granulated sugar

• 2 large eggs, at room temperature

• 1 tablespoon vanilla extract

• 1 cup (227g) sourdough starter, unfed/discard

• 2 cups (241g) King Arthur Unbleached All-Purpose Flour

• 1 tablespoon potato flour or 2 tablespoons instant mashed potato flakes

- 1 teaspoon baking powder
- 1/2 teaspoon baking soda
- 1/2 teaspoon salt
- 1/4 cup (57g) milk, at room temperature
- confectioners' sugar, optional

Instructions:

- Preheat the oven to 350°F. Grease a 9" square pan.
- To make the topping: In a medium bowl, whisk together the flour, sugar, cinnamon, and salt. Add the vanilla and almond extracts to the melted butter and pour the butter into the flour mixture, stirring until you have a uniformly moist mixture. Set aside while you make the batter.
- To make the batter: In a large mixing bowl, beat the butter and sugar until well combined. Add the eggs, vanilla, and starter, mixing until smooth and scraping the bowl's sides and bottom as you go.
- In a medium bowl, whisk together the all-purpose flour, potato flour, baking soda, salt, and baking powder. Add to the butter/starter mixture, stirring until evenly combined. Add the milk and mix until smooth.
- Spread the batter in the prepared pan. Sprinkle the crumb mixture evenly over the top.

• Bake the cake for 45 to 50 minutes, until a paring knife inserted in the center comes out clean, and the edge of the cake just barely pulls away from the pan. Remove it from the oven and cool on a rack; dust the top with confectioners' sugar.

• Store the cake, the pan covered with plastic, at room temperature for several days; freeze for longer storage.

Sourdough Chocolate Chip Cookies

Ingredients:

• 2 cups all-purpose flour (310g)

• 1 tsp baking soda (6g)

• 1/2 tsp salt (4g)

• 3/4 cup butter (170g) melted

• 3/4 cup sugar (160g)

• 3/4 cup brown sugar (120g)

• 2 eggs

• 1/2 cup sourdough starter discard (160g) 2-5 days old

• 1 tsp vanilla (5g)

• 2 cups chocolate chips (340g)

Directions:

- Preheat oven to 350°F.

- Stir flour, baking soda, and salt together in a medium mixing bowl; set aside. *If at high-altitude, also add 3/4 tsp baking powder. See high-altitude modifications in post above.*

- In a large mixing bowl, beat butter, sugar and brown sugar on medium-high speed until light and fluffy.

- Mix in eggs, one at a time, until incorporated. Add vanilla and sourdough starter discard; mix well. Some separation is normal at this stage.

- Slowly add flour mixture to wet ingredients, and mix until just incorporated. Add chocolate chips and stir in by hand using a spatula.

- Prepare a cookie sheet by greasing with oil or butter, or lining with silpat or parchment paper.

- Drop 12 teaspoonful of dough onto the cookie sheet, maintaining a consistent size and spacing evenly apart.

- Bake 9-12 minutes, until starting to turn golden on edges. Remove from oven and allow to sit on cookie sheet for 5 minutes, then transfer to a cooling rack with a lifter.

- Repeat for remaining cookies.

• Freeze any uncooked dough as instructed above in post.

Classic Sourdough Banana Bread

Ingredients:

• 1/3 cup softened butter

• 1 cup white sugar

• 1 teaspoon vanilla

• 1 egg

• 3 bananas mashed

• 1 cup discard sourdough starter stirred

• 1 ½ cups all-purpose flour

• ¼ teaspoon salt

• 1 teaspoon baking powder

• ½ teaspoon baking soda

Instructions:

• Preheat oven to 350. Prepare a loaf pan by greasing with vegetable oil spray or butter.

• Beat the butter and sugar in a large mixing bowl with an electric mixer on medium speed. Add the egg and vanilla, mixing until combined. Add the mashed banana and sourdough starter, mixing on low.

• In a separate medium mixing bowl mix the flour, salt, baking soda, and baking powder. Add it to the wet ingredients and mix on low until just combined.

• Pour into loaf pan, smoothing out the top with a spatula, and bake in preheated oven for 1 hour, or until a toothpick comes out clean. The top will split. Allow to cool before slicing. Store at room temperature, tightly wrapped, for up to three days.

Soft and Moist Sourdough Zucchini Bread

Ingredients:

• 3 cups all-purpose flour

• 1 tsp salt

• 1 tsp baking powder

• 1 tsp baking soda

• 1 tbsp cinnamon

• 3 eggs

• 4 tbsp sourdough discard* see notes

• 1 cup vegetable oil

• 1 1/4 cups sugar

• 3 tsp vanilla extract

• 2 cups grated zucchini do not drain or remove moisture

Instructions:

- Preheat oven to 325°F. Grease two 8×4" pans.

- In a medium bowl, stir together the flour, salt, baking soda, baking powder and cinnamon. Set aside.

- In a large bowl, beat eggs, sourdough discard, oil, vanilla and sugar. Slowly add dry ingredients to wet ingredients and mix well. Add zucchini and stir until incorporated.

- Pour batter into prepared pans, about half in each. Bake 45-60 minutes, or until tester or butter knife inserted in the center comes out clean. Cool in pans for 15 minutes, then remove loaves onto cooling rack to cool completely.

Sourdough chocolate chip cookies

Ingredients:

- 1/2 cup sourdough starter

- 1/2 cup butter, softened or coconut oil

- 1 to 1-1/3 cups flour

- 2/3 cup granulated cane sugar

- 1 egg

- 1 teaspoon vanilla extract

- 1/2 teaspoon sea salt

- 1 teaspoon baking soda
- 1/2 teaspoon baking powder
- chocolate chunks, dried fruit, or crispy nuts (optional)

Instructions:

- In a medium sized bowl, combine sourdough starter and butter.
- Add one cup of flour. Mix well. Continue adding flour a little at a time, mixing well after each addition, until you get a very stiff dough.
- Cover with a kitchen towel and allow to sour at room temperature for 8 or more hours.
- Preheat your oven to 375 °F and get your baking sheet ready. Grease the baking sheet or line with parchment paper.
- Mix egg, sugar, vanilla, sea salt and baking powder in a separate bowl. (Hold the baking soda for a bit.)
- Pour the egg mixture over the top of your soured dough. Blend well (I use my hands).
- When dough is well mixed, add chocolate, fruit, etc, blend thoroughly. Lastly, sprinkle the baking soda over the top and mix well.

- Drop by spoonfuls onto a cookie sheet. Bake for 10 to 12 minutes, until bottoms are lightly brown and tops are soft set.

- Cool completely on a wire rack. Store in an airtight container with wax paper between layers.

- Makes around 2-3 dozen cookies, depending on the size.

Sourdough Blueberry Crumb Cake

Ingredients:

- Crumble Topping

- 1/4 cup (50g) sugar

- 1/2 cup (100g) light brown sugar

- 1 1/2 cups (180g) all-purpose flour, spooned and leveled

- Rounded 1/2 tsp cinnamon (use 1 tsp for more flavor)

- Pinch of fine sea salt

- 8 tbsp or 1 stick (113 g) salted butter, cut into small cubes, cold

Wet Ingredients

- 8 tbsp or 1 stick (113 g) salted butter

- 1 cup (200 g) sugar

• 1 large egg

• 1/2 cup (120g) leftover sourdough starter discard (see note below)

Dry Ingredients

• 2 cups (240 g) all-purpose flour, spooned and leveled

• 1 tsp. baking powder

• 1/2 tsp baking soda

• Pinch of fine sea salt

• 1/2 cup (120g) sour cream

• 1 heaping cup of fresh blueberries

• Powdered sugar

Directions:

• Preheat the oven to 350 F. Lightly oil an 8×8-inch pan and line with parchment paper. Smooth the bottom and sides of the pan so the paper is flat.

• Add the blueberries to a small bowl. Sift a tablespoon of powdered sugar over the top and gently toss to combine. This will prevent the berries from sinking into the cake. Set aside.

• To make the crumble topping, add all of the ingredients to a medium-sized bowl. Mix into crumbles using your hands. The butter should be well blended into to the flour; some larger pieces are ok. If using frozen crumble topping, remove it from the freezer now.

• In a small skillet, melt the butter until light golden brown around the edges (you are not fully browning the butter). This will only take a few minutes, but do not walk away from the pan- it will burn quickly!

• Meanwhile, using a stand mixer, beat the sugar, egg, and sourdough starter on medium-low speed, 1 minute. With the machine running, gradually pour in the warm melted butter.

• In a separate bowl, sift the dry ingredients. Add to the wet ingredients and mix on low speed until just combined. You should still see specks of flour in the bowl; do not over mix. Add the sour cream and mix until smooth. This technique will give the cake a soft, velvety texture. The batter will be thick.

• Spoon the batter into the pan. In an even layer, scatter some of the crumbles over the top first, then do a layer of blueberries. Repeat to finish all of the crumbles and blueberries. See my note on this below.

• Bake for 55-65 minutes or until a toothpick comes out clean when inserted (I use a dried piece of spaghetti). Please check at the 50 minute mark to see how things are going.

• Cool completely before serving. Dust with powdered sugar.

Sourdough Scones with Blackberries & Lemony Glaze

Ingredients:

Scones:

• 2 cup fresh or frozen blackberries (or raspberries or other berries)

• 2 1/2 cups all-purpose flour (see notes)

• zest from one lemon

• 1/2 teaspoon salt

• 1 1/2 tsp baking powder

• 1/2 teaspoon baking soda

• 1/2 cup sugar

• 1/2 cup cold butter- sliced into 8 pieces (or vegan butter)

• 1 cup sourdough starter (275 grams)

• 1/3 cup milk or cream (or nut milk, plus more if necessary)

• 1 beaten egg, for brushing, optional

Lemony Glaze:

- 1/4 cup Fresh Lemon Juice
- 1 cup powdered Sugar
- 1 tablespoon butter (optional)
- Garnish with more lemon zest if you like.

Instructions:

- Line an 8-inch cake pan with parchment and fill with 2 cups fresh berries. If your berries are very tender, freeze for 30-60 minutes beforehand, this way they will hold their shape (and not smash) a little better.

- In a food processor, pulse flour, lemon zest, salt, baking powder, baking soda and sugar. Pulse in cold butter until mixture resembles coarse sand.

- In a small bowl mix milk and sourdough starter together. Add the starter mixture to the food processor and pulse until it just forms a ball (just a few times) adding a little more milk only if necessary. Dough should be heavy and thick. Don't overwork it.

- Spread the dough over the berries and press down gently, into all the corners with your fingers. Place in the freezer for 2 hours.

- Preheat oven to 400F. Remove dough from the freezer and invert on cutting board. Let sit a few minutes or longer until thawed enough to cut. Cut into 8 equal size pie shape wedges. Brush with beaten egg (optional). Space them 2 inches apart (they will puff and spread a bit) on parchment-lined baking sheet, let thaw 20-30 minutes and bake for 25 minutes or until golden brown.

• While baking, make the glaze. Stir sugar into lemon juice in a small pot on the stove until dissolved. Whisk in butter (optional). Set aside. Drizzle over warm scones.

Sourdough Brownies

Ingredients:

• 150g (5.3 ounces) dark chocolate (65-70% cocoa solids)

• 50g (1/4 cup) unsalted butter

• 60g (1/4 cup) vegetable oil

• 2 eggs + 1 egg white (if you're in Europe use size 'large'. If you're in the US use size 'extra-large')

• 1/2 tsp salt

• 150g (2/3 cup) caster sugar or granulated sugar

• 110g (1/2 cup, packed) light brown sugar

• 2 tbsp water

• 1 tsp vanilla extract

• 50g (1/2 cup) unsweetened cocoa powder

• 120g (1/2 cup + 2 tbsp) sourdough starter (100% hydration) (see notes)

Instructions:

• Preheat the oven to 180°C/375°F fan. Line a 7.5 x 9.75-inch (19 x 25 cm) rectangular or 9-inch (23cm) square brownie pan with baking paper.

• Break the chocolate up into chunks. Place into a medium pot with the butter and vegetable oil. Set over a low heat on the stove and stir often (to prevent it burning), until the chocolate is almost fully melted. Remove from the heat and set aside so the remaining chocolate can melt from the residual heat.

• This next step can be done in a stand mixer with the whisk attachment, or in a large bowl with electric beaters: Place the eggs, egg white, salt and both kinds of sugar into a large bowl (or the bowl of the stand mixer) and whisk until pale and very fluffy. Add the water and vanilla then continue to whisk until the sugar has mostly dissolved - you can tell when this has happened by rubbing some of the mixture between your fingertips, if it feels very grainy, you need to keep whisking. This will take about 10-15 minutes.

- Mix the cocoa powder and sourdough starter into the melted chocolate mixture until completely combined.

- Add this mixture to the bowl of whipped egg mixture and fold together until just combined.

- Pour into the prepared brownie tin and bake for 30-35 minutes (SEE NOTES). The top should look dry and a toothpick inserted into the centre of the brownies should come out with a little bit of batter still stuck to it, but not LOADS.

- Let the brownies cool for at least 20 minutes before slicing into 16. Sprinkle with some flaky salt if you want!

Sourdough Discard Pumpkin Bread Recipe

Ingredients:

- 1 2/3 cups all-purpose flour
- 1 teaspoon baking soda
- ¾ teaspoon baking powder
- 1/4 teaspoon salt
- 3 teaspoons pumpkin spice
- 3 large eggs room temperature
- 2/3 cup coconut oil (or your favorite mild flavored oil)
- 1 cup sugar
- 1 cup unfed sourdough starter room temperature
- 1 teaspoon vanilla extract
- 1 cup canned pumpkin puree not pumpkin pie filling

Candied pepita topping

- 1/3 cup pepitas pumpkin seeds
- 1 teaspoon honey
- 1/2 teaspoon coconut oil or any mild flavored oil

Instructions:

• Preheat the oven to 350°F. Line 9x5 loaf pan with parchment paper and spray with baking spray (or butter and flour the pan).

• Combine the dry ingredients in a large bowl. Whisk to combine the ingredients and set aside. In a separate large bowl, combine the eggs and whisk well. Add the oil, sugar, starter and vanilla. Stir until it is all combined. Add the pumpkin and mix until incorporated. Use a spatula to get all the ingredients from the side of the bowl and combine them.

• As soon as you prep batter, prep the candied pepitas (pumpkin seeds). There are two ways to make it: you could heat up the pumpkin seeds with the honey and oil in a small skillet until it is combined, OR if you have a microwave, microwave it for 10 seconds to melt the honey and help it combine easier.

• Transfer batter to prepared pan. Smooth the top and sprinkle the candied pepitas (pumpkin seeds) over the top.

• Bake for 55-65 minutes or until toothpick inserted into the center of the loaf comes out clean (every oven is different. We baked ours for about 65 minutes). If getting too brown, cover lightly with foil after 45 minutes. For the smaller pans bake for about 25-30 minutes.

• Cool for 20 minutes, then slide out of pan and transfer to a cool rack. Cool completely before slicing.

Sourdough Waffles

Ingredients:

The Night Before

• 2 cups all purpose flour (300g) preferably unbleached

• 2 cups buttermilk (475g)

• 2 tbsp sugar (30g)

• 3/4 cup sourdough starter discard (215g) unfed

• The Morning Of

• entire overnight sponge

• 1/4 cup butter (55g) melted

• 2 large eggs

• 3/4 tsp salt

• 1 tsp baking soda

• 1 tsp cinnamon optional

• 1 tsp vanilla extract optional

Instructions:

The Night Before

• Overnight sponge: stir the unfed starter discard and measure out 3/4 cup (215g). In a large bowl, stir together the flour, sugar, buttermilk and the 3/4 cup (215g) starter.

• Cover with a kitchen towel and leave on counter overnight, letting the sponge rest at a room temperature between 65°F – 70°F overnight, or 12 hours.

The Morning Of

• In the morning, start by preheating your waffle iron. Peek at your sponge and see how much it grew! (Older kids love this part.)

• Beat together the butter and eggs in a small bowl. Stir into the overnight sponge.

• Add the salt, baking soda and optional ingredients if using, and stir to combine. You'll notice the batter start to produce bubbles – this is how you know it's ready!

• Spray cooking oil on your preheated waffle iron and pour batter onto the plate. Close the lid and bake according to manufacturer's recommendations.

• When waffles are done, remove with silicone tongs and serve immediately, or place on cooling rack, to guarantee crispness.

Tip: Place a cooling rack on a baking sheet in a warm oven to hold your waffles as you cook the remainder. This will allow air to circulate around the waffles, preventing them from becoming soggy on the bottom.

Tip: To freeze, allow to cool completely on cooling rack, then stack and place in freezer bags. Parchment paper in between waffles is optional, but not necessary. Reheat in microwave or toaster.

Simple Sourdough Bread Recipe

Think sourdough bread is too complicated to bake at home? Think twice! This sourdough bread recipe is so easy & simple that I promise you will want to bake it again and again! It's delicious, frugal & healthy, plus there's no kneading required!

A freshly baked crusty sourdough boule sitting on top of a striped tea towel. The text overlay reads Simple Sourdough Bread.

I also love it because:

• Making bread from scratch is one of the healthiest and most frugal ways to save money on food.

• All you need for sourdough is a starter, whole wheat flour, a pinch of salt, and some water!

• You can even make a gluten-free starter and adapt this recipe for gluten-free sourdough bread!

Ingredients:

• A half-full jar of einkorn sourdough starter culture with a spoon stirring the culture. The jar is sitting on top of a striped tea towel.

• Sourdough Starter. Sourdough bread needs an active starter culture (which is made of beneficial bacteria and yeast) to create the sour flavor of the bread. You can make your own sourdough starter from scratch (or get a sourdough kit to help speed along the process).

Homemade Buffalo Wing Sauce

This sourdough bread recipe needs to have an active starter culture, but if you don't have any currently, here is my post for tips on the sourdough starter. Whole Wheat Flour. You can use white flour if you don't have whole wheat or are not comfortable using whole wheat in baking yet. It may be easier to experiment with the lesser expensive flour and once you've found your sourdough groove, upgrade to whole wheat. Here are some tips on the dough:

You want to bake with a starter that is at its peak – when nearly all of the yeast has eaten but hasn't begun to go dormant because of the lack of food. You can see when a starter has peaked because it will have a dome-shape on top.

Starters peak in the 2-3 hour range after each feeding.

• Don't skimp on the water that recipes call for. Sourdough recipes are wetter than traditional bread recipes made with baker's yeast.

• The press-your-thumb-to-test-for-springiness test works. Do it.

• The see-through-your-dough test works too. Try it.

• Two rises will produce a more sour bread than a single rise.

• I use a bread proofing basket called a "banneton" to let my sourdough bread rise. I use this kind here.

• A complete list of ingredients with the amounts you need is located in the recipe card below.

Step-by-step instructions

A jar of sourdough starter culture is ready to be used in this sourdough bread recipe. The half-full jar sits on top of a kitchen tea towel, beside a clean silver spoon.

Here's how to make this sourdough bread recipe from scratch.

• Step 1: In a very large bowl, mix the sourdough starter, water, and 3 cups of whole wheat flour with a wooden spoon and combine well.

• Step 2: Add salt and remaining flour 1/2 cup at a time, attempting to completely stir in the flour with each addition. When you can no longer mix with a spoon, use your hands to mix in the flour. Continue adding flour until your dough begins to resemble dough, but is still sticky and “pourable.”

• Step 3: Pour the dough into a banneton (I like this one) and fill 1/3 way up. Cover with a towel and allow it to sit in a warm place for 4-12 hours, until the dough is at least doubled in size and looks to be “domed” on top. The fresh sourdough dough has risen to double its size, and is now ready to be baked in a Dutch oven or 2 loaf pans.

• Step 4: When the dough is at least doubled in size, flip the banneton over so that the dough dumps directly into a Dutch oven, lined with parchment paper, (or loaf pans). If the dough doesn’t come out centered into the Dutch oven pot / loaf pans, wait 20 seconds, then grab the handles and shake the dough so it’s centered.

• Step 5: Place the Dutch oven or loaves in a cold oven and turn the oven on to 350 degrees. Bake bread for 50-60 minutes, until the edges are golden and the bottom sounds hollow when tapped

• Step 6: Remove to cool on wire racks for at least 30 minutes.

www.ingramcontent.com/pod-product-compliance
Lightning Source LLC
LaVergne TN
LVHW021307160826
845679LV00001B/244

* 9 7 9 8 3 6 4 6 1 2 1 2 0 *